30-DAY WATER ENEMA THERAPY

The Most Powerful Method to Prevent & Cure Diseases

By- Ayurvedic Practitioner

Chander Kant Singh

Copyright © 2019 Chander Kant Singh

All rights reserved.

Table of Contents

Introduction 6

Chapter 1: History of the Water Enema 10

Chapter 2: Importance of a 30-Day Water Enema Therapy 12

   How Our Intestines Work 12

   Bowel Movements & Intestines 13

   The Very First Symptom of Digestive Issues 14

   Toxins in the Body 15

   Natural Way to Clean & Heal the Body Internally 17

Chapter 3: How to do a 30-Day Water Enema Therapy 19

   30-Day Water Enema Therapy to Prevent Disease 19

   30-Day Water Enema Therapy to Cure Disease. 21

Chapter 4: The Therapeutic Benefits of a 30-Day Water Enema Therapy 23

   Constipation 24

   Liver Detox 26

   Intestinal Parasites 27

Irritable Bowel Syndrome (IBS) 28

Leaky Gut Syndrome 29

Food Allergies & Sensitivities 29

Skin Condition 30

Indigestion 31

Migraine 31

Insomnia 32

Bad Breath & White Tongue 33

Malnutrition 33

Obesity 34

Chronic Sinusitis 34

Arthritis 35

Disease Prevention 35

Chapter 5: How to Prepare Yourself for a 30-Day Water Enema Therapy 37

Importance of Fasting 37

Use of Herbal Medicine 38

Overcoming Food Addiction 38

Starting Organic Food 38

Importance of Mono Meal 39

Chapter 6: How to Do a Water Enema 41

Distilled Water is Best 41

Cold & Lukewarm Water Enema 41

Quantity of Water to Use 42

Method & Steps to Follow 42

Chapter 7: Herbal Supplements to Heal the Intestines 44

Green Juice of Herbs & Vegetables 44

Quercetin 44

Probiotics 45

Chapter 8: Herbal Remedies for Intestinal Parasites Cleanse 46

Black Walnut 46

Cloves 46

Ginger 47

Garlic 47

Recipe to Kill & Remove Intestinal Worms 47

Chapter 9: Side Effects of Water Enema 49

When to avoid a 30-Day Water Enema Therapy 49

Chapter 10: Myths about Water Enema 51

Loss of Electrolytes 51

Loss of Peristaltic Movements 51

Loss of Gut Flora 52

Chapter 11: Testimonials 53

Obesity, High Cholesterol & Digestive Issues 53

Digestive Health, Sinusitis & Hair loss 53

Parasite Cleanse & Water Enema 54

Chapter 12: FAQs 55

Introduction

The *30-Day Water Enema Therapy* book is going to be your best friend to keep you healthy. A daily water enema continuously for 30 days is the most powerful way to prevent and cure disease. Ayurveda believes that the root cause of most diseases is unhealthy gut and keeping it healthy can be a matter of life or death. Water enema is the only way to wash the most toxic part of the digestive system. The therapeutic health benefits of water enema make it an important part of the world's oldest Indian traditional health care system known as "*Ayurveda*".

There are many diseases which are difficult to cure. Medicine can or cannot cure the disease due to their limited effect and many times they are ineffective. The human body knows the self-healing process and we only need to provide the right environment to make it happen. After applying water enema therapy on many patients and on myself for 4 years, I have been able to develop a complete treatment that can prevent and cure diseases. It is divided into two parts. The first part helps to prevent the disease and its progress, and the second part helps to cure the disease. There are important and different steps to be followed for the success of the therapy. These steps involve the use of water enema, a unique type of fasting and diet which are essential for detoxing and healing the body from inside to prevent & cure the disease. This is a unique therapy which can be used independently or in combination with any medical system to cure any disease.

This book provides thorough knowledge and understanding to do this therapy yourself for your health and wellbeing. It provides complete and detailed information in a step-by-step manner about this therapy for health professionals, students, and patients. This *30-Day Water Enema Therapy* is simple, safe, and easy to perform at home.

This book is dedicated to my family and to the memory of my grandfather, Shri Jameet Thakur, who passed away due to lung cancer. I want to thank you, the reader and congratulate you in advance for buying this book.

About the Author

Chander Kant Singh graduated as a Bachelor of Ayurvedic Medicine and Surgery from Mahaganpati Ayurvedic Medical College Affiliated by Rajiv Gandhi University of Health Sciences Bangalore. His education continued at the University of Aberdeen in Scotland where he received his master's degree in International Health Care and Management. He is a registered Ayurvedic Practitioner by Ayurvedic and Unani Medicine Board in India.

Disclaimer

This book is a combination of information taken from ancient Ayurvedic texts and experience acquired through Ayurvedic practice in India. This book is for information and educational purpose only and cannot be taken as medical advice. The author cannot be held responsible for any adverse effects that may arise from the use of this treatment. You must Consult an Ayurvedic practitioner to start the Water enema Therapy.

Copyright

This book is copyrighted by Chander Kant Singh and no person has the right to reprint or resell this book. No part of this publication may be reproduced in any form or by any mechanical means, including storage in a retrieval system or transmitted in any form without permission in writing from the publisher.

Copyright © 2019 Chander Kant Singh

All rights reserved.

Chapter 1: History of the Water Enema

In Ayurveda, water is known as "Jal" and enema is called "Basti". Using water for an enema has been a universal practice since ancient times. We call it simply "Jal Basti", and it is an ancient yogic practice with many benefits for the body and mind. The ancient Indian medical system, also known as Ayurveda, is one of the world's oldest medical systems. Its aim is to cure disease naturally and to protect the health of a currently healthy person. Water enemas are used as an important tool to cure many diseases even today. It is believed that the root of most diseases is the unhealthy large intestine, which is also called the colon. It is the most toxic part of our body and it is recommended to use an enema in ayurveda to keep it clean.

The colon is the place for "vata" dosha according to Ayurveda. Vata is one of the three basic pillars of our body. It is responsible for the movement in the mind and the body. All the activities take place in the body due to the vata. Every disease originates from the imbalance of vata dosha. It controls the elimination of wastes in the body and helps in breathing, blood circulation, and movements of the body.

Keeping the colon clean keeps the vata in its place and leads to a healthy and disease-free life. If we review this even from the modern point of view, the above facts are still true in many ways. The large intestine is the part of the human digestive system that stores and eliminates fecal matter. An unhealthy colon has an adverse effect on our health, and it becomes the root cause of almost every disease that can be treated just by keeping it healthy. An enema effectively washes the toxins from the colon which are the root cause of every disease. The effect of an enema on our health and quality of life is not limited to only the colon, but it is much more than we think.

Chapter 2: Importance of a 30-Day Water Enema Therapy

Water enema has several health benefits that start from the colon and spread throughout the body in a step-by-step manner. Minimum of 30 days are required to achieve the therapeutic effects of this therapy. A perfectly working digestive system is key to maintaining a healthy body and mind. A small change in its function makes a big difference in the way we feel because it affects the whole body. A strong immune system is directly linked to a clean colon. The human gastrointestinal tract is made up of the oral cavity, esophagus, stomach, liver, pancreas, gallbladder, small intestine, large intestine, and anus. To understand the importance of *30-Day Water Enema Therapy,* it is important to know about the intestines, where the direct and indirect effects of the water enema take place.

How Our Intestines Work

Human intestines are divided into two parts known as small and large intestines. The small intestine is composed of three parts: duodenum, jejunum, and ileum. Food gets digested by the secretions of the digestive juices in the small intestine and then nutrients get absorbed. Next is the large intestine, which is composed of three parts: cecum, colon, and rectum. Cecum is the first part of the large intestine that joins to the last part of the small intestine. The second part is the colon, and it is further divided into four parts: ascending colon, transverse colon, descending colon, and sigmoid colon. The third part is called the rectum. Our colon is designed to absorb water and nutrients from food and to create stool. The next function is to remove the waste and toxins from the body regularly. This way, the body gets detoxified automatically every day. Our intestines are continuously working, and that's the reason they are very vascular. They use a lot of energy to digest every food particle. The colon is five feet long and has a very efficient blood supply. It is connected to veins that drain it, and it merges with the portal vein that goes back to the liver.

Bowel Movements & Intestines

Modern science still has not been able to reach the deepest part of our small intestinal tract, due to its length and shape, which acts as a physical barrier. This barrier makes it impossible for us to see what is happening inside the intestines daily. It takes a very long time to recognize health issues that arise from here. Any change in bowel movement always has a relationship to the digestive system itself. Intestines do special contraction and relaxation movements known as "peristalsis", which moves the food from the small intestine to large intestine for digestion and the elimination process. These peristaltic movements are continuing in the small intestine to digest food and in the large intestine to absorb water and nutrients and to store stool in the rectum. Everyone has a different pattern of bowel movements because it depends on the individual's diet and lifestyle. As a result of these bowel movements, many people expel stool daily, and some do not have that in days. Normally, we eat three meals in a day and stool should be eliminated three times as well, but hardly does anyone passes three stools daily.

The Very First Symptom of Digestive Issues

Most of the time, the first common symptom of a digestive issue is constipation, whereas gas, bloating, abdominal cramps, and acid reflux are also there. Any digestive problem with or without the above symptoms must be taken seriously because it can become the basis of an unhealthy life. Digestive problems can change bowel movements. If waste is not expelled on time, it makes the colon walls "encrusted", thereby making it difficult to perform its job. From here toxins are absorbed by the colon and carried back into the liver, which is called "autointoxication". A body may get poisoned by toxic substances that are not eliminated. This can cause an overgrowth of bacteria and fungi, which can enter the small intestine and lead to an inflammatory reaction in the lining of the whole intestine. Such a situation over the long-term triggers leaky gut syndrome and related problems like irritable bowel syndrome (IBS), stomachache, swelling, indigestion, fatigue, worms, intestinal obstruction, allergies, bloating, candidiasis, food cravings, lethargy, body odor, making us feel sluggish and heavy. This effect is not limited just here it can further reach our vital organs. It can become the cause of serious illness like cancer.

Toxins in the Body

Toxins are the harmful substances that are of two types: exotoxins and endotoxins. These days, human beings are constantly getting exposure to exotoxins. These toxins are present in the air, water, and food. Use of pesticides, insecticides, chemicals, and pollution are the main sources of external toxins. Endotoxins are those which are produced inside of the body. In the human body, maximum toxins are produced and expelled out of the body through the large intestine where stool is formed from the digestion of food. The next is the toxins produced at the cellular level through the metabolic process. The liver is the only organ that detoxifies all kinds of toxins. It changes them into less toxic form and throws it into the intestine in the form of bile for the digestion of food. In the end, it becomes the job of the colon to expel the maximum amount of toxins from the body. This clearly shows that the colon is the most toxic part of the body. Moreover, intestinal parasites are the sources of the toxins that are constantly circulating in the body. Toxins are always the root cause of diseases. When these toxins are not expelled from the body, they start to build up and produce symptoms and in later stage create a disease. To prevent a disease, it is important to wash the colon daily to remove the toxins which are present inside the colon. To cure a disease, the first step is to remove the toxins from the liver & body tissues and secondly heal the body. This can be done with the help of a special method of doing enema, fasting and taking a new diet. We can understand clearly that the aim of the treatment must be detoxification and healing.

Natural Way to Clean & Heal the Body Internally

The human body has self-healing mechanism. In Ayurveda, healing process is always encroached upon with the use of natural methods. If these methods fail to cure independently, then the use of herbs and some herbal formulations is recommended. It is always advised to use fresh herbs because of their strong healing powers. Most of these herbs are used in our daily life. Some common examples are mint, coriander, spring onions, parsley, and basil. These herbs help clean and heal the body.

For proper healing, the human body needs energy and rest. As we know, our maximum energy is spent in the process of digesting food. When we allow the digestive system to rest, it boosts the healing process.

We all clean our mouth daily to keep us healthy. Similarly, it's a basic need of our body to clean the end part of the digestive system regularly. In *30-Day Water Enema Therapy,* toxins are expelled from the body. The special method of fasting and change in diet help heal the body. During this time period, our digestive system gets enough time to clean, heal and remove toxins.

Stool formation is a continuous process and it must be eliminated on time. Water enema removes both the fresh and old deposits of stool. This process helps detox the whole intestine. It also removes the intestinal parasites and prevents their growth. Elimination of toxic material daily prevents the progress of many diseases. It makes the immune system strong enough to keep the body healthy and disease-free and this approach can cure any disease.

Chapter 3: How to do a 30-Day Water Enema Therapy

There are few steps involved in a *30-Day Water Enema Therapy*. These steps must be followed in a proper manner to do it correctly. This therapy is divided into two parts. The first part involves the process to prevent the disease and its progress. The second part involves the process to cure the disease. The minimum length of the therapy is 30 days which cures many diseases. However, it can be continued even after 30 days to cure a disease or health issue.

30-Day Water Enema Therapy to Prevent Disease

Prevent a Disease: Many people want to keep themselves healthy and disease-free. Preservation of good health is a challenge in the modern world where food, water, and the environment are toxic. It is necessary to remove the toxins from the body and to keep our digestive system clean to stay away from the diseases. Here, water enema therapy is a very effective and natural way that can preserve the health of a healthy person. It is recommended to do water enema twice daily for a period of 30 days. It must be done in the morning and in the night before bedtime. Although no further steps are required, it is recommended to add more salad, fruit, and vegetables to the diet to prevent the accumulation of toxins in the body. Water enema can be repeated for 30 days once a year to keep you clean internally which is the key factor for preserving good health

Prevent the Progress of a Disease: There are many diseases which are incurable, and it is important to stop their progress to preserve the health. Water enema therapy is a very effective and natural way to do it. Here are the three steps that can be easily followed. It is possible that a disease starts to cure while following this process. This process of water enema must be followed for a minimum of 30 days and it can be repeated whenever it is required to control a disease.

First Step: The first step is to do water enema twice a day for 30 days. It must be done in the morning and then in the night before bedtime. This step remains the same for the whole *30-Day Water Enema Therapy*.

Second Step: This step involves the diet. It is important to change your diet and introduce salad, fruit, and vegetables. Reduce the amount of cooked food in your diet because it has more toxins. You can enjoy your favorite cooked meal once a day. It is best to take it in the afternoon or at night. It keeps you satisfied and prevents the progress of diseases.

30-Day Water Enema Therapy to Cure Disease

There are three important steps to follow to cure any disease. This process can be followed by anyone who wants to cure themselves of any disease.

First Step: The first step is to do water enema twice a day for 30 days. It must be done in the morning and then in the night before bedtime. This step remains the same for whole *30-Dyas Water Enema Therapy*.

Second Step: The second step is to do fasting and in ayurveda, it is also known as *"langhan chikitsa"*. This is a unique type of fasting that must be done every day for a specific time. This dry fasting starts in the morning and continues for 6 to 8 hours. During this time, do not eat or drink anything. This gives enough time for the body to heal & cure its health problem. This process must be continued for 30 days along with the use of water enema. Many patients feel thirsty in the morning and they cannot stay thirsty. Drinking water stops the process of natural healing because the body starts to digest the water. Here, water enema plays an important role. This method does not stop the natural healing because it bypasses the mouth & stomach. It hydrates the body and satisfies the urge of thirst for 6 to 8 hours.

Third Step: This step starts with breaking the dry fast every day. This must be done with the help of a green juice. Diet is an important part of this step to cure a disease. Eat raw food like fruits, vegetables, and salad in the afternoon. Reduce the amount of grains, pulses, meat, egg and stop alcohol during this treatment. You can have your favorite meal for dinner. The first aim of this diet is to reduce the formation of toxins and to save the energy for the healing process. Liquid diet has very less amount of toxins but solid foods like grains and pulses have more toxins and body spends a lot of energy to process such food. The second aim of this diet is to reduce the amount of fecal matter which is toxic to our body and becomes food for the intestinal parasites.

Note: While doing dry fast for 6 to 8 hours, it is important to avoid any medicine. Take medicine after this time because medicine also stops the process of detoxification & healing. It is also good to complete your medicine course or stop it temporarily according to the need.

Chapter 4: The Therapeutic Benefits of a 30-Day Water Enema Therapy

A water enema has numerous therapeutic health benefits. Anyone having a healthy colon can live a natural, healthy, and disease-free life until old age. If your colon is kept clean, you never need to see a doctor. It is the best natural way to detox and cleanse the liver, intestines, and the body. The unique quality of the water enema is that it can be used in any disease while taking any medicine. It gives instant and long-lasting results in many diseases. It can be used along with any detox and weight loss program to boost the results. Nowadays, it has gained so much importance that people do it at home with the home enema kit. During these 30 days, several things take place inside the body, and that gives enough time to gain therapeutic benefits. Here are the key benefits of *30-Day Water Enema Therapy*.

Note: The therapeutic effect of this therapy is not limited to the diseases that are explained below. It can be done for any disease to cure it completely. These are some common examples where we can use this treatment.

Constipation

As we know, the colon is the main part of the digestive tract that holds the most toxic material in the body. Here is the base location for many diseases to start and to end as well. Constipation is a condition where stool is not eliminated on time. It is the first symptom from which a disease gets a root cause to start. People around the world suffer from this problem, but they never think that it can lead to a serious health effect on their life.

The people around the world spend a lot of money for many medicines to get rid of constipation. These medicines are easy to take because of their shape in the form of pills and liquids. Many of these give good results in the beginning but become ineffective in later stages. The reason is that these medicines only cure the symptoms, but not the cause of the problem. These mostly work by extracting water from the blood supply of the intestines through the lymphatic system to expel the fecal matter; in addition, some increase the peristaltic movements to get it done. This process causes fluid loss in the body, along with the loss of vital nutrients, which becomes the reason for the weakness in the body often felt by such patients. The second fact is that taking laxative medicines and remedies has a negative effect on the health of our intestines and makes them weak if taken for long periods on a regular basis. Thirdly, these medicines prevent the absorption of digested food, which leads to many nutritional deficiencies. Finally, these medicines have a greater toxic effect on our body than benefits, such as habitual usage of these medicines, digestive issues, and liver and kidney damage. In order to cure constipation in this manner, we are doing more harm to our health, wealth, and quality of life instead of having any long-term benefit.

When we think about the 30-day water enema therapy, it is a different story. The first, most immediate effect of the water enema is to remove constipation. The way it works is safe and natural in approach. In the enema, water is supplied externally, and it does not interfere with the blood supply of the intestines. Secondly, it improves the strength of the intestine by helping it to remove toxic material. Third, it does not interfere with regular digestion of food because the enema has its effect in the large intestine.

Here, water supplied with the enema process softens the hard stool and breaks it into smaller parts. While this action takes place, the large intestine starts the process of expelling it. It takes 10-15 minutes to clear the last part of the intestine. This makes enough room for the stool that is stuck behind to move forward. A four-week continuous water enema removes all the old stool deposited inside and makes it normal to come out every day on time. To get rid of constipation, it is important to introduce the water enema and stop the use of laxatives once the constipation is relieved.

Liver Detox

The liver is the second largest organ of the body. It is the chemical hub because it deals with all the toxins that are absorbed by the intestine and it changes them into a less toxic form. Accumulation of toxins can disable the liver and disturbs the normal function of the whole body. It can lead to digestive problems and other health issues. The liver is connected to the intestine with the portal vein. The large intestine absorbs the water and nutrients and sends them to the liver by the portal vein. A water enema keeps the intestine clean and indirectly reduces the amount of toxins supplied to the liver. It prevents the reabsorption of the toxins and prevents autointoxication. When a water enema is done continuously, it gives a break to the liver to do its functions properly. This leads to a boost in the digestion and the functioning of the liver. Fasting and diet boost the detoxification and healing process of the liver. A simple liver function test, done before and after the course of the *30-Day Water Enema Therapy*, clearly shows the improvement in the liver function.

Intestinal Parasites

There are many types of intestinal parasites such as roundworms, pinworms, bacteria, viruses, fungi, and candida that live in the digestive system. These parasites release a lot of toxins that never let our body clean and heal. It is necessary to get rid of them to prevent and cure any disease. *30-Day Water Enema Therapy* helps to cure this problem. Here, cold-water enema is excellent to kill worms that live inside the last part of the digestive tract. The reason is the temperature change inside the intestine. Worms cannot keep themselves warm, and cold water kills them instantly. An enema also takes away the fecal matter that gives shelter to these organisms. Toxins that arise due to the dead worms can cause a lot of health issues, and a water enema prevents this situation by eliminating them along with their toxins. The water enema allows the intestine to heal and regain its strength. It provides a healthy environment to host good bacteria and unfavorable conditions to the parasites.

To get rid of intestinal worms that live inside the small intestine, it is recommended to use some herbal formulations as described in chapter number 8. Following the whole treatment regularly for 30 days gives a complete cure.

Irritable Bowel Syndrome (IBS)

This is a common condition related to the digestive system that everyone encounters once or many times, at any stage of life. There are many known and unknown reasons for this health problem. Food allergies, food intolerance, intestinal parasites, overgrowth of intestinal bacteria, constipation, and indigestion are the common causes. In Ayurveda, IBS is considered as "Aam", and it means indigestion. The first step is to find out the list of foods that you are allergic to or intolerant of with the help of an igE "immunoglobulin" blood test. Doing a *30-Day Water Enema Therapy* improves the digestion and cures indigestion by removing toxins and healing the intestine. Taking a probiotic to introduce a new healthy gut flora while doing the enema for 30 days helps re-establish good bacteria, and it is recommended to use some herbs to heal the intestine as described in chapter number 7.

Leaky Gut Syndrome

This is a health condition where the intestinal inner lining becomes damaged. It increases intestinal permeability. This causes many types of infections and health issues. There are many reasons for leaky gut syndrome. The common causes are intestinal parasites, food allergies, use of drugs, inorganic and processed food. A *30-Day Water Enema Therapy* helps get rid of the parasites and the bad bacteria that cause leaky gut syndrome. It creates an environment inside the digestive system that allows the intestine to heal and regain its strength. It is important to avoid the food and medicines that trigger leaky gut. It is best to use herbs to clean and heal the gut as described in chapter number 7 & 8.

Food Allergies & Sensitivities

This health condition is linked to the immune system. It can be genetic, such as a wheat allergy or celiac disease and acquired due to a change in the immune response. There are many elements that trigger the immune system to respond incorrectly towards food. These may include the presence of intestinal worms, medication, chemicals, pesticides, preservatives, and infection. Under any conditions, it is beneficial to know the food items that you are allergic to and are causing constant damage to your health. A simple igE "immunoglobulin" test can help here. Such allergy-causing foods should be avoided for a period of one month from the start of the *30-Day Water Enema Therapy* which helps us recover from food allergies and sensitivities. It is important to clean and heal the intestine to recover the health and immunity power. Again, it is recommended to use herbs and formulations as described in chapters 7 & 8.

Skin Condition

The skin is the largest organ of the body. Its function is to protect our body and to eliminate toxins. When the toxic load in the liver increases beyond its capacity, it expels these toxins to the skin to increase the detoxification process. The skin is unable to detox a lot of toxins and starts to develop health issues. There are many skin problems that start to develop such as rashes, dermatitis, skin allergies, vitiligo, dark circles under the eyes, dry or oily skin, psoriasis, hair loss, and early signs of old age. Human skin and the intestine are closely linked together. The primary source of these toxins is food that is not processed properly and stays inside the colon for a longer duration than normal. The only way to remove this toxicity is to perform a *30-Day Water Enema Therapy*. It improves the skin condition quickly and skin becomes normal, healthy, and glowing within a few days.

Indigestion

Many people suffer from chronic indigestion, which is called "Aam" in Ayurveda. When we have such problems, it becomes difficult to keep yourself active and healthy. More often, a congested colon, disabled liver, and gallbladder make the digestion process slow and incomplete. This results in the production of more toxic substances. It makes the digestive system inefficient, causing bloating, acid reflux, burping, cramping, and constipation. A complete *30-Day Water Enema Therapy* becomes helpful to re-establish the healthy environment within the liver and intestines thereby improving the digestion of the food and absorption of the nutrients.

Migraine

Headaches are a common sign of dehydration, constipation, and toxicity in the body. These are mostly linked to the digestive system. Dehydration can be easily cured by taking more fluids and water. People who suffer from dehydration also have constipation. Again, a congested colon has a link to headaches. A water enema plays a very important role here to help cure the headache. There is a considerable improvement in the headaches soon after doing the water enema. There is a feeling of lightheadedness, mental clarity, a boost in energy, and relaxed mind. The reason is the elimination of the toxic material from the colon and improved hydration of the body. This is the instant health benefit, and to prevent the migraine completely, it is important to do a *30-Day Water Enema Therapy*. According to Ayurveda, pain in the head is the symptom of vata disease and its origin is in the colon. Water enema keeps the colon clean and improves the hydration level and improves blood circulation. This provides more energy to the brain and detoxifies it. This is a key health benefit, which makes the water enema an important tool to cure migraines. It helps stop the use of many unnecessary medicines.

Insomnia

Insomnia is a health condition where sleep is disturbed. In our modern society, we have become sleep-deprived, and it has increased the stress level in our daily lives. Lack of sleep has many negative effects on our body and mind. It keeps our energy level low and depresses the body functions. In Ayurveda, sleep is called "nidra", and it is considered one of the three pillars of our life. If sleep is disturbed, then it has long-term serious effects on our health. The human brain needs proper sleep to remove its toxins to function properly. When we have health issues related to our digestion like indigestion, gas, intestinal parasites, constipation, or other digestive issues, it increases the toxicity in the body. An accumulation of toxins has a direct effect on our sleep patterns. Here, the *30-Day Water Enema Therapy* gives great relief. It removes the unwanted toxic substances from the body and helps cure the underlying health condition, and when the toxic load decreases from our body, it relaxes the nervous system and induces sleep.

Bad Breath & White Tongue

Bad breath indicates an increase in bacterial activity, and white tongue is a symptom of indigestion. It can be due to bacterial overgrowth, intestinal worms, constipation, food allergies, or poor oral hygiene. Poor digestion causes rotting of undigested food and production of more toxins in the body. This causes bad breath and a white coating on the tongue. Doing a *30-Day Water Enema Therapy* removes the toxins and improves the digestion.

Malnutrition

Malnutrition in the body can also be due to improper digestion or poor absorption of the digested food. If our digestive system is unable to work normally, then the nourishment is reduced to the body. This decrease in nourishment causes tiredness and lethargy, which make the body physically weak. Here *30-Day Water Enema Therapy* makes the intestine strong and healthy. This improves the digestion of food and absorption of the nutrients.

Obesity

Obesity is a disease where the weight of the body increases due to the deposition of fat tissue more than the normal amount. It can be due to taking extra calories in the diet or due to a health condition. A *30-Day Water Enema Therapy* helps reduce the weight. The diet and dry fasting involved in this treatment reduce the calories intake. Moreover, an enema removes the built-in fecal matter, which also provides instant weight loss. Here, diet, fasting, and enema combined provide excellent results.

Chronic Sinusitis

Chronic inflammation in the sinus causes this condition, and there are many reasons for it. Mostly, allergic reactions or underlying digestive health problems have a link to it. Nasal congestion, headaches, bad breath, fever, and insomnia can be associated with this problem, and these symptoms get worse when indigestion is experienced. It has a negative effect on health in the long-term, so it is important to start a proper *30-Day Water Enema Therapy*. Once the intestine and digestive system start to work normally, the sinusitis itself gets cured. Removal of toxins and promotion of healing boost the immunity power and help the body to cure sinusitis. It helps stop the unnecessary medication and promotes a healthy lifestyle.

Arthritis

This is a health condition where joints are painful. It can be osteoarthritis, rheumatoid arthritis or gouty arthritis. Ayurveda says the origin of the arthritis is from the improper digestion and accumulation of toxins in the body tissues. To cure this disease, it is important to follow a complete *30-Day Water Enema Therapy*. This improves the digestion and removes the toxins from the body ultimately curing the disease.

Disease Prevention

Water enema removes and prevents the buildup of toxins in the intestine, liver, and body tissues. According to Ayurveda, the large intestine is the place of vata dosha, and keeping this organ unhealthy becomes the root cause of many illnesses. Keeping it clean boosts the immunity power and makes the body strong and healthy. In this way, it creates a healthy environment, which stops the development of new diseases. That is the reason *30-Day Water Enema Therapy* is helpful to maintain good health.

Chapter 5: How to Prepare Yourself for a 30-Day Water Enema Therapy

A *30-Day Water Enema Therapy* gives an opportunity to start a new healthy life. It is essential to prepare yourself for this treatment. Many people can start it straight away without any problem. However, some need time to start it. It is best to spend some time preparing yourself mentally and physically for the water enema, fasting and changing the diet. All these steps are explained below in detail.

Importance of Fasting

In Ayurveda, fasting means avoiding food and water for some time to cure a disease. Dry fasting for a minimum of 6 hours is not difficult, many people can do it easily; however, it is recommended to do some practice for those who are new to this process, before starting a *30-Day Water Enema*. It is best to do some dry fast that starts from the morning along with an enema. It keeps the body hydrated and prevents the urge of thirst. Always break your fast with a green juice. Try to extend the time of dry fasting day-by-day to 6 hours. Once you can do it, you are ready to start the actual process of *30-Day Water Enema Therapy*.

Use of Herbal Medicine

Herbal medicines are natural and more beneficial to cure disease. Ayurvedic medicines are herbal in nature, and these medicines improve the repair and development of new cells in the body. It is important to replace your medication with herbal medicines to promote a good environment inside your body. However, there are many medicines that have no alternative, and they may be essential for health. In such conditions, continue your present medicine. You can consult an herbal or Ayurvedic doctor to start these medicines as an alternative to your regular medicine. These medicines improve the immune system and help the body to recover naturally.

Overcoming Food Addiction

Food is a basic need of our body to survive, but over time, many food items become our addiction, which is not healthy at all. It is always difficult to overcome this problem, so it is recommended to replace it with a healthy diet slowly. It is best to take 7 to 10 days to do this. While doing water enema and dry fasting, your body easily adapts to the new diet.

Starting Organic Food

In Ayurveda, food is considered a medicine. If food is taken wisely, then we can prevent and cure many diseases without any medicine, so diet is an important part of this treatment and should be taken seriously. It is important to stop eating inorganically grown food, processed food like refined flour and sugar, fried food, fast food, meat, and dairy products. Change your diet to an organically grown plant-based diet that includes green leafy vegetables, fruits, and salads. The water inside the fruits and vegetables is so nourishing that it makes your overall health better than before. To get maximum nutrition out of a salad, it must be chewed properly and slowly. The amount of salad that should be taken is according to body weight. Take two percent of your body weight in salad. Always eat food that is easy to digest. Cooked food should be avoided but it may be difficult for some people. Here, cooking must be done on slow heat so that it preserves the nutrients. Slow cooking is best, and the use of slow cooker is an excellent example. It increases the nutritional value and taste of the food. It also reduces the amount of toxins produced inside the body after digestion.

Importance of Mono Meal

A mono meal means a meal with only one type of food. For a mono meal, you can choose any vegetable or fruit or boiled grain, for example, eating only watermelon as a breakfast meal until you satisfy your hunger. There are many benefits of taking a mono meal. It helps the digestive system to digest the food easily without using much energy. The intestines can absorb nutrients more efficiently, and fewer toxins are produced. It improves the digestion and healing of the intestine.

Chapter 6: How to Do a Water Enema

It is important to keep a positive approach towards this process as we are doing it to help our body. Follow the instructions and steps properly as described below to achieve your goal towards a healthy life.

Distilled Water is Best

Water is a universal solvent. It dissolves toxins when used in an enema and cleans the large intestine. The safest and most effective type of water is in the distilled form. It is free from infection and gives maximum benefits. Hence, it is used in the medical field for many purposes. Distilled water produced by a home water distiller is also a good choice, as the distiller can be used anytime. Filtered water can be used as an alternative to distilled water and it must be used after boiling. It makes it hygienic to use for the enema process.

Cold & Lukewarm Water Enema

Both cold and lukewarm water can be used for *30-Day Water Enema Therapy*. It is recommended to use cold water for enema that is at room temperature and should be between 25 to 35 degrees Celsius. It is beneficial to kill the intestinal worms that are present inside our digestive tract. Lukewarm water can be used in the first few days to make you comfortable.

Quantity of Water to Use

The maximum amount of water that can be used for one complete enema process without stressing your body is 1 to 1.5 liters. This amount is enough to gain health benefits. In *30-Day Water Enema Therapy,* two enemas are recommended, one in the morning and one in the night. Take 1 to 1.5 liters of water each time.

Method & Steps to Follow

When ready to do the enema, just fill the enema bag and hang it or place it at a height equal to your chest. Now, it is very important to run the water off into the bath or sink to get rid of air bubbles to avoid any inconvenience. There is an on/off tap at the end of the long tube. Now, lie down on your right side with your knees slightly up towards the chest or make a body position like a dog by touching your knees and forearms on the floor and lower your front portion down and keep your hips high. Apply some coconut oil to the end part of the tube and your anus. Try to insert the nozzle slowly into your anus and do not push it hard. Insert it at a 90-degree angle straight in and let it go inside easily. Once the nozzle is inside, turn on the tap and allow the water to go in and turn off the tap and remove the nozzle out slowly when you feel to do so. Try to hold the water inside you as long as you can easily do it. Once you feel the desire to expel the water, just do it and then relax for a couple of minutes. Now repeat the process again and you should be able to finish the water in 2 to 3 attempts. If you feel uncomfortable to finish the water, then just discard the remaining water. You may feel two to four motions in the whole process and these motions stop themselves.

Chapter 7: Herbal Supplements to Heal the Intestines

While doing a *30-Day Water Enema Therapy*, it is helpful to use some natural supplements to heal the inner walls of the intestines. These supplements are optional to use with the enema process. These enhance the healing property of the whole treatment.

Green Juice of Herbs & Vegetables

In Ayurveda green juice is also known as "swaras". It is a fresh extract of the leaves extracted with any method like the use of mortar & pestle or a machine. There are many ways to prepare it and its flavor and taste can be enhanced with the use of salt and pepper. Use fresh herbs like ginger, mint, basil, parsley, coriander, and any other green herb available. It is good to add a small quantity of herbal extract or leaves to carrot, sweet pepper or any other vegetable that is available to make the juice. This green juice is very effective to boost the healing and detoxification process.

Quercetin

Quercetin is a plant-based dietary supplement that helps the intestine to heal quickly. It takes around six weeks for the intestine to generate a new gut lining. Quercetin blocks the tiny holes and provides enough time for healing and regeneration of new intestinal cells. Quercetin is a plant flavonoid that is found in many fruits, vegetables, leaves, and grains. You should take 500mg of capsules or tablets twice a day after food continuously for30 days. The most common vegetables and fruits that contain high amounts of quercetin are red onions, peppers, black grapes, kale, asparagus, broccoli, and tomatoes.

Probiotics

Water enema removes both the good and bad bacteria that live in our colon, and it is important to increase the number of good bacteria after the treatment. These microorganisms boost the healing process of the intestine and control the growth of the bad bacteria. It is best to introduce a good probiotic supplement for 30 days.

Chapter 8: Herbal Remedies for Intestinal Parasites Cleanse

Water enema alone cannot kill and remove all the intestinal parasites, but it provides an opportunity to get rid of them. It is recommended to take some herbal medicines while doing water enema for a month. The most effective herbs that are used in ayurveda against the parasites are explained below.

Black Walnut

This plant has developed strong protection for its seeds and nuts. The useful part of this tree is its green hull of black walnut. It has many potent chemicals, herbicides, fungicides, and vermicides which kill the parasites that are adults or in their development stage. It is recommended to add 500mg of black walnut power into your water enema. It kills the worms instantly.

Cloves

These are excellent to eliminate parasite eggs by destroying their outer covering. Cloves are the only herb that kills the parasites' eggs. They can be used in herbal tea or in a juice. Take one to two cloves once daily. In Ayurveda, cloves are commonly used in the preparation of many anthelmintic medicines.

Ginger
This is an herb and can be simply added to food and juice. It kills the worms and their larva at any stage of their life cycle. It must be a part of the diet. It can be taken daily for 30 days, and it enhances digestion, liver function, and bowel movement.

Garlic
Garlic is commonly used in many food items to enhance their flavor and taste. It is beneficial for overall health. It not only kills the worms but is also effective against bacteria, virus, fungi, and parasites. Eating garlic in high doses is not recommended because it can lead to gastritis and digestive upset. Just add one or two cloves of garlic to your diet.

Recipe to Kill & Remove Intestinal Worms
Take 30 grams of mint leaves, 10 milliliters fresh lemon juice, black pepper powder or seeds 1 gram, 500mg black walnut powder, and some salt. Put all these ingredients into a mixer and make a paste. Keep it in a bowl and take 2 to 4 teaspoons of it at the time you break your dry fast during the enema therapy. Take it with water or a drink made up of yogurt. It is easy to make a drink of yogurt. Just add 200ml water to 3 to 4 spoons of yogurt and mix it to make a milky solution. This is a great recipe that kills

and removes the worms of any kind that lives inside our digestive tract. Take it continuously for 3 to 4 days.

Chapter 9: Side Effects of Water Enema

A water enema has no side effects if it is done in a safe and proper manner. People are doing it without any issues. The side effects that happen are when a water enema is done during a serious illness, using contaminated water, or an accidental tear is made inside the colon. While following the proper procedure, such side effects are never experienced. People fear putting water inside the rectum because they do not know about it. They believe it is not natural to do or it is not a comfortable thing to do. However, anyone who does it the first time can believe that the truth is totally different. It gives instant relief from many health issues.

When to avoid a 30-Day Water Enema Therapy

There are certain health conditions in which it is not a good idea to start a water enema without medical supervision. Water enema is not recommended in pregnancy, dysentery, rectal bleeding, menstruation, extreme weakness and any condition that can cause harm. It is always best to ask your doctor if you have doubts regarding your health issues before performing the enema.

Chapter 10: Myths about Water Enema

Many people believe that water enema is unhealthy and unsafe. It is assumed that it can cause loss of electrolytes, loss of peristaltic movements, damage to the gut flora, and weakness in the body. However, all these claims are made by those people who never did a water enema in their life or lack of proper knowledge about it. A proper water enema does all the opposite to the claims made above.

Loss of Electrolytes

The first claim is the loss of electrolytes, which never happens because the water in a water enema is supplied externally, and our colon is not forced to drain water and electrolytes from its blood supply. This water does not stay inside for a long time. It comes out within a few minutes and it never comes out in the same amount. It is always less in quantity because our colon absorbs a small amount of it to clear the dehydration.

Loss of Peristaltic Movements

The second claim is that it causes loss of peristaltic movements. Here, we are doing a water enema to cure constipation and to remove old fecal matter, which should not be there in the first place. Having such health issues means that peristaltic movements are already improper. When a water enema is done, it helps the intestine to expel this old toxic matter. Once the colon gets cleared, our intestine has less work to do and it gains its strength and normal function. After doing it for four weeks, bowel movements become normal and constipation or any related health issues get cured.

Loss of Gut Flora

The third common claim is the damage to the gut flora. We are doing a water enema because we have some health issues related to our digestive system. That means we already have an imbalance of gut flora. There are more bad bacteria there. Here, a water enema removes all these good and bad bacteria from the large intestine and mainly from the last parts of it. Water only reaches the sigmoid colon and rectum; it never goes deep inside the large intestine and small intestine. This means that only a small portion of the intestine is involved here. Hence, it is not possible to have a loss of gut flora from the whole intestine.

Chapter 11: Testimonials

Obesity, High Cholesterol & Digestive Issues

A patient aged 46 years old did a *30-Day Water Enema* to cure many health issues. She had obesity, high cholesterol, heartburn, indigestion, and constipation. She had blood pressure around 270/90 most of the time.

Her starting weight was 77 kg, and at the end of the treatment, she was 69 kg. She passed dead worms in her enema process. Her symptoms were improving daily. After one month, her blood cholesterol level was normal. There were no digestive issues and her blood pressure was normal around 126/84. She was disease-free and was able to live healthy without medicine.

Digestive Health, Sinusitis & Hair loss

One of my patients did *30-Day Water Enema Therapy* to recover from digestive issues, sinusitis and hair loss. She was a 36-year-old female, and she was taking medicines for all these health issues.

She passed dead parasites (roundworms) during this treatment. The water enema was continued for a total of 30 days. After that, she had improved digestion with no sinusitis symptoms and hair loss completely stopped. She was not on any medication after this. Her skin started to glow and was looking much healthier than before.

Parasite Cleanse & Water Enema

A male patient aged 35 years had weight 49 kg, celiac disease, indigestion, chronic diarrhea, many food allergies and sensitivities, and roundworms infection. He was taking medicine for almost every disease listed above. He eventually did *30-Day Water Enema Therapy*.

The patient was physically weak due to his poor health condition. He eliminated a lot of dead parasites with each water enema. He continued the water enema daily for 30 days. It improved the intestinal strength and he was physically more active than before. He had better digestion and was able to eat more types of food than before. His chronic diarrhea went away, and his sleep pattern improved. He did not need any supplements or digestive medicines after the one-month period and his weight increased every month. After three months, his body weight was 55 kg.

Chapter 12: FAQs

Is water enema safe or not?

Water enema has been done for thousands of years in India and is considered the healthiest way to keep you healthy.

Can a water enema remove the mucous lining of the colon?

A distilled water enema does not cause harm to the mucous lining of the large intestine. When an enema is done, you can see there is no such thing coming out with the water.

Are there any side effects to doing an enema daily for 30 days?

There are no side effects to doing a water enema daily. It will not cause any negative effect on the natural bowel system, but it will make it healthier. It is a common practice in yogic science and in Ayurvedic treatments.

Can a regular enema cause loss of peristaltic movement?

Doing an enema for four weeks continuously and then according to need cannot cause this situation. We are doing a kind of mini-water enema daily where the quantity of water is less and according to comfort. This amount of water has no side effects.

What kind of lubricants should be used?

Olive oil and coconut oil are the best oils to use for lubrication of the nozzle and anal region.

Can I use salt and oils as enema liquids?

Do not try to add anything to the enema water. It can have side effects. Be patient and do it with distilled water to see the positive changes. Using anything else should be done only under the supervision of a doctor.

Is water enema the same as Basti in Ayurveda?

A water enema is a kind of Basti. The actual Basti is only done by the Ayurvedic Panchakarma Specialist with the use of medicated oils and ghee.

Can a water enema be used in children?

It is not recommended to do this without the supervision of a doctor. A small mistake can cause serious harm to the child. The biggest risk is to tear the rectal wall with the nozzle. Only trained nurses or medical professionals know how to administer an enema to children.

Can a daily enema kill all the gut flora?

Our intestine is a long, tube-like structure. The water enema can only reach the last part of the large intestine. The complete removal of the gut flora with the water enema is not possible. The length of the large intestine is 4 to 5 feet whereas the enema water can travel only 1 to 2 feet and peristaltic movements push it out within a few seconds to a few minutes. Moreover, when we have problems in our intestines, there are more bad bacteria in number than good bacteria. Removing them gives a good opportunity to replace them with healthy gut bacteria by taking a good prebiotic daily.

How many bowel movements are normal after a water enema?

Two to four bowel movements will take place normally as the intestine will try to remove this water.

Can a water enema damage the colon?

A water enema makes the colon healthy. It prevents and cures many diseases. The only way a colon gets damaged is with physical force and the wrong method of inserting the nozzle of the enema bag. It is important to take care while doing an enema and to never force the nozzle while inserting it inside.

Can an enema cause dehydration?

No, a proper water enema never causes dehydration because it makes the colon hydrated and it never extracts water from the intestine. A water enema works with the water that is supplied externally, and some water gets absorbed by the colon which helps to rehydrate the body.

Can water enema cause electrolyte issues?

Again, a water enema never causes electrolyte imbalance in the body if done properly. The reason behind this is that water is supplied externally and we do not lose any water from our body in this process. Water stays inside the colon for only a few minutes, and it just breaks down the fecal matter and comes out. It cannot go inside the colon wall and take out the electrolytes.

Can you get addicted to an enema?

No, you cannot get an addiction of water enema. It can be done safely for a few months. It helps the digestive system to improve its function.

Can a nozzle dilate the anus and cause permanent issues with it?

We have never experienced this happening so far. The nozzle is very small in size and goes inside the anus smoothly. It is made for this purpose, and within the recommended size and shape it is safe to use.

How often should the enema kit be changed?

Do not use an enema kit for more than a month. It is best to buy enema kits that are reusable for easy replacement. There can be a chance of infection building inside the nozzle or the tube. It is always the best practice to keep it clean and wash it after every use.

Does the 30-day water enema cure any disease?

When a water enema is done as a healing process for four weeks, it gives enough time for the body to regain its capability to heal faster. It removes the toxic material from the intestines, liver tissues, and skin. Anyone who does it for even the first day can say that it works. A complete *30-Day Water Enema Therapy* can prevent and cure many diseases. However, it depends on many factors, so the best is to try it and see how much benefit you get.

Is a daily enema safe to do?

It is an ancient practice to do an enema daily by both yogic and the people who follow Ayurveda. The amount of water used here is small, and only two enemas are done daily. This kind of enema does not put stress on our system, and it is safe to do.

Should I consult a doctor before doing a water enema if I have a disease?

It is best to check with your doctor so that they can suggest to you if it is safe to do while suffering from a disease. There are certain medical conditions in which it can be dangerous to do it.

Can I help someone to do a water enema?

If you know the procedure and the person who wants to do it has no knowledge about it, then you can assist him in the water enema process. Usually, people do a water enema themselves once they understand the whole process. After doing it once, it becomes easy to do it alone the next time you want to do it.

I am not able to do 6-hour dry fasting what should I do?

It can be done with practice. It is better to do dry fasting for a few hours every day and increase the time slowly.

I am always thirsty in the early morning, what should I do?

It is better to drink enough liquids during the day and evening time. You can drink water in the middle of the night but avoid in the early morning. Do water enema in the morning when you feel thirsty, this will hydrate you immediately and you can feel that within a few minutes.

How long can I follow Water Enema Therapy?

This therapy is safe to perform for a longer duration. It can be easily done for 2 to 3 months. Water enema can be stopped after 1 month and diet can be followed for next months. It can be done accordingly but water enema is a must for the first 30 days.

Can I eat fried and cooked food?

Eating fried food occasionally is not bad. Cooked food must be cooked on slow fire to prevent the formation of toxins. It is advised to do minimum cooking and use a slow cooker or crockpot for cooking purpose.

Can I make any kind of green juice?

There are endless ways to make green juice. Just make the one you like but avoid adding sugar to it. Just add salt, pepper or herbs to the juice.

Can I do water enema once a day only?

Yes, you can do that but that reduces the effect of the therapy; however, it is still effective.

Can I skip a few days of water enema?

You can do that but do it regularly and do for a total of 30 days as soon as possible.

My disease is cured, should I stop this therapy?

Congratulations on your success! You can stop the regular use of water enema and fasting but do it whenever you feel like doing it. Keep a healthy diet to stay healthy.

www.ingramcontent.com/pod-product-compliance
Lightning Source LLC
Chambersburg PA
CBHW072207170526
45158CB00004BB/1787